Best Foreplay Guide for Sexual Pleasure

25+ Top Foreplay Tips, Tricks and Ideas You'll Be Dying to Try

Cheryl Bach

Best Foreplay Guide for Sexual Pleasure

©2024 by Cheryl Bach

Publisher: IntimateInk Press

Email: intimateinkpress@gmail.com

This book is a work of nonfiction intended for informational purposes only. The content of this book is based on the author's research, knowledge, and experience, and it is provided with the understanding that the author and publisher are not engaged in rendering legal, medical, or professional advice. The information in this book is not a substitute for professional guidance or assistance. Readers should consult with relevant professionals for advice and assistance regarding their specific situations. The author and publisher disclaim any liability for any loss or risk, personal or otherwise, which is incurred as a consequence, directly or indirectly, of the use and application of any of the contents of this book.

Cover design by IntimateInk Press

Interior layout and design by IntimateInk Press

Printed in USA

Fonts: Google fonts

Image: Freepik.com. This cover has been designed using assets from Freepik.com

For permission to use copyrighted material from this book, please contact the copyright holder listed above.

First Edition: 2024

Distributed by Amazon.com, Inc.

Cheryl Bach

Table of Contents

Cheryl Bach

Chapter I
Introduction

Foreplay is easily one of the most important aspects of sexual activity. It is the ideal way to get both partners in the right frame of mind and heighten arousal before getting intimate. A truly satisfying sexual experience should include plenty of foreplay.

Benefits of Foreplay

Foreplay has immense benefits that help build strong relationships and keep them steamy for longer:

Enhances emotional and physical intimacy: By communicating with your partner about what works and what doesn't, you can create a sense of deeper understanding and intimacy between you.

Helps you relax: Since foreplay begins long before actual sex, it gives you time to relax into each other and really enjoy yourself.

Better preparedness: good foreplay helps you prepare for and ease any discomfort during further sexual activity.

Increased arousal: Both partners need to be fully aroused to enjoy sexual activity, and foreplay is an excellent way to get there.

Allows you to explore your partner's body and preferences: Each person's body and preferences are unique, trying out new things with your partner is a great way to explore and learn what you like together.

Cheryl Bach

By understanding the importance of foreplay and its role in building a strong emotional and physical bond with your partner, you can add a new level of intimacy and excitement to your sexual life.

In the following chapters of this book, we will explore over 25 top tips, tricks and ideas on how to master foreplay and experience more pleasure. From understanding the types of foreplay, to exploring erogenous zones, kissing techniques and more, you'll have everything you need to become a pro at foreplay and truly satisfy your partner's desires.

Foreplay is not just about physical touch, it also involves verbal and emotional connection. Seductive whispers, flirtatious texts, and teasing banter are all part of the experience. It's about building a strong bond not just physically, but emotionally as well.

We will also discuss how you can avoid common mistakes that can ruin the mood. Understanding what drives men and women wild, and what to avoid during foreplay, is crucial for a successful session. Knowing how to create a safe environment for open communication, and how to prioritize pleasure for both partners, will strengthen the bond between you.

So get ready to explore new techniques and try new things together. You'll be amazed at how much more satisfying your sexual experiences can become with just a little extra attention to foreplay.

Finally, it's important to emphasize that foreplay is not just something you do to kill time before the "real" action starts. Foreplay is an integral part of sexual activity and shouldn't be overlooked or rushed. It's a way to build trust, intimacy, and excitement between partners. Whether you're kissing, touching, tickling, or whispering sweet nothings, foreplay can be a fun and enjoyable experience for both people involved.

Remember, Communication and consent are essential for good foreplay. Take the time to listen to your partner and explore their desires. This guide will help you develop your skills and techniques, but it's up to you and your partner to find what works best for you.

We understand that everyone is unique, and what works for one couple may not work for another. That's why we encourage experimentation and trying out new things. Stay open to new experiences and be willing to explore different techniques. By incorporating these ideas into your foreplay routine, you will discover new levels of pleasure and intimacy with your partner.

In conclusion, there's no denying the importance and benefits of foreplay in a romantic relationship. It's an essential building block of sexual activity, creating emotional and physical connection between partners. With the right mindset, communication, and techniques, foreplay can be a fun and enjoyable experience for everyone involved. So, get ready to take your foreplay game to the next level and experience new heights of pleasure and intimacy with your partner in the coming chapters of this book. Thanks for reading, and we hope you find this guide helpful as you explore the world of foreplay!

Chapter II
Types of Foreplay

Foreplay is not a one-size-fits-all affair. There are different types of foreplay, each designed to stimulate and arouse your partner in unique ways. In this chapter, we'll explore the three major types of foreplay - physical touch, verbal communication, and sensual teasing - and how to use them to maximize pleasure and intimacy in your relationship.

Physical Touch

Physical touch is probably the most well-known type of foreplay. It involves using your hands, mouth, and body to stimulate your partner's erogenous zones. The goal is to build arousal and desire by slowly exploring your partner's body, alternating between gentle and firm touches.

Here are some techniques:

Start with light touches: Begin by lightly stroking your partner's arms, legs, back, and neck. This helps to create a sense of anticipation and builds excitement.

Mix it up: Don't limit yourself to one type of touch. Use a combination of gentle caresses, deep pressure massages, and teasing tickles to keep your partner on their toes.

Explore erogenous zones: Take your time to find out what areas of your partner's body are particularly sensitive. These could include the neck, ears, breasts, thighs, and genitals. Pay attention to how your partner responds to different types of touch.

Cheryl Bach

Verbal Communication

While physical touch is important, it's not the only way to increase arousal and build intimacy during foreplay. Verbal communication can be equally stimulating, especially when done in a seductive and flirtatious tone.

Here are some techniques:

Soft whispers: Whispering sweet nothings into your partner's ear can be incredibly arousing. Tell them how much you desire them, describe what you want to do to them, or recount your past sexual experiences together.

Dirty talk: If your partner is up for it, incorporate some dirty talk into your foreplay routine. This could involve describing in detail what you want to do to them, or using explicit language to express your desires.

Compliments: Complimenting your partner's appearance or sexual abilities can also be a turn-on. Let them know how sexy and desirable they are.

Sensual Teasing

Sensual teasing involves getting your partner's anticipation and desire levels up by teasing them in a non-physical, but still provocative way.

Here are some techniques:

Eye contact: Eye contact can be incredibly seductive, so maintain steady eye contact with your partner during foreplay to build intimacy and increase arousal.

Dress up and slow strip: Dressing up in sexy outfits and performing a slow strip tease for your partner can be a fun way to build anticipation. Make sure to use music and lighting to create a sensual atmosphere.

Cheryl Bach

Delayed gratification: Tease your partner by slowly building up to the main event. Take things slow and focus on building tension and anticipation. This could include teasing touches, dirty talk, and sensual kissing.

Bonus Tip: Incorporate Props

In addition to these three types of foreplay, you could also incorporate props to make the experience even more exciting and pleasurable. This could involve using toys, blindfolds, or even food items.

Whatever type of foreplay you choose, make sure to communicate openly with your partner about your desires and boundaries. Building trust and intimacy through foreplay is essential for a healthy sexual relationship, so take the time to explore and experiment with different techniques until you find what works best for both of you.

In conclusion, foreplay is an essential part of any sexual encounter. By incorporating different types of foreplay, such as physical touch, verbal communication, and sensual teasing, you can build arousal, anticipation, and intimacy with your partner, paving the way for a more enjoyable and fulfilling sexual experience. So go ahead and try out some of these tips, tricks, and ideas - you'll be amazed at the results!

Chapter III
Techniques for Physical Touch

Physical touch is an important part of foreplay that can really get both partners in the mood. But it's not just about random touching - there are techniques you can use to make touching more pleasurable and exciting. In this chapter, we'll explore some of the best techniques for physical touch, including kissing, caressing and stroking, mutual massage, direct stimulation of erogenous zones, and oral sex tips and techniques.

Kissing Techniques

Kissing is one of the most intimate forms of physical touch and a great way to start off foreplay.

Here are some kissing techniques to try:

Start slow: Begin with light kisses on the lips, then gradually begin to lick and suck on your partner's lips.

Nibble the earlobe: The earlobes are a sensitive erogenous zone for many people. Try lightly nibbling on your partner's earlobes while you kiss.

French kiss: To add more passion to your kissing, use your tongue and lightly explore your partner's mouth with it.

Mix it up: Don't just stick to kissing on the lips - try kissing their neck, ears, and other sensitive areas to add variety to your make-out session.

Cheryl Bach

Use different pressures: Experiment with soft and gentle kisses, as well as deeper, more passionate ones. Varying the pressure can keep things interesting.

Caressing and Stroking

Caressing and stroking are tactile techniques that involve using your hands to sensually touch your partner's body.

Here are some tips:

Use different textures: Experiment with different textures, like soft fabrics or feathers, to enhance the sensation of your touch and make it more pleasurable.

Explore the body: Focus on exploring different parts of your partner's body, like their shoulders, arms, chest, and back. Gradually work your way down to more intimate areas.

Vary the pressure: Use light, feathery touches to tease your partner, or apply firmer pressure for a more intense sensation.

Use your whole hand, not just your fingers: Use your palm, fingertips, and even the back of your hand to caress and stroke your partner's body.

Mutual Massage

Massages are a great way to relieve stress and tension, but they can also be a powerful tool for foreplay.

Here are some tips for mutual massage:

Use massage oil: Massage oil or lotion can add a sensual element to your massage and make it feel more pleasurable for both partners.

Focus on erogenous zones: Pay special attention to your partner's erogenous zones, like the neck, ears, and inner thighs.

Use different strokes: Try different massage techniques, like effleurage (light, sweeping strokes), petrissage (kneading), and friction (circular motions).

Don't forget the feet: Massaging your partner's feet can also be a surprisingly sensual experience that can help relax them and set the mood for more intimate activities.

Direct Stimulation of Erogenous Zones

Direct stimulation of erogenous zones is a great way to build arousal and anticipation during foreplay.

Here are some tips:

Use your fingertips: Use light, teasing touches on sensitive areas like the nipples, clitoris, and penis.

Vary the sensation: Experiment with different sensations by using your fingertips or a toy to provide light touches, firm pressure, or vibration.

Focus on the whole body: Don't just focus on the more obvious erogenous zones - explore other areas of your partner's body, like the inner thighs, back of the knees, and even the ears and neck.

Pay attention to your partner's cues: Watch for their reactions and listen to their feedback to gauge what feels good for them.

Oral Sex Tips and Techniques

Oral sex can be an incredibly pleasurable experience for both partners, but it can also be intimidating if you don't know what you're doing.

Here are some tips:

Communicate with your partner: Ask them what they like and what feels good, and be open to feedback.

Experiment with different techniques: Try different ways of using your tongue and lips, like using circular motions or varying your pressure.

Focus on the clitoris: The clitoris is a highly sensitive area, so pay close attention to it. Use your tongue or fingers to provide direct stimulation.

Don't forget about his/her penis/balls: Just like with the clitoris, use your tongue and lips to provide direct stimulation to your partner's penis or balls.

Mix it up: Try different positions and techniques, like 69 position or using your hands in addition to your mouth.

In conclusion, there are many techniques for physical touch that can help make foreplay more pleasurable and exciting. Experiment with different techniques and remember to communicate with your partner to find out what feels good for them. By doing so, you'll be well on your way to a more satisfying and intimate sexual experience.

Chapter IV
Techniques for Verbal Communication

Physical touch is an incredibly important aspect of foreplay, but it's not the only one. Verbal communication can also be a powerful tool for building intimacy and arousal. In this chapter, we'll explore some techniques for using words to enhance your foreplay experience.

Flirty Texts and Sexting

In today's digital age, there are more ways than ever to communicate with your partner. Flirty texts and sexting can be a fun and exciting way to build anticipation and set the mood for your next intimate encounter.

Here are some tips:

Use playful language: Experiment with puns, emojis, and other playful language to add a lighthearted and flirtatious tone to your messages.

Start off slow: Don't jump right into graphic descriptions of what you want to do to your partner. Build up the anticipation by starting with suggestive messages that hint at what's to come.

Be specific: Use specific language to describe what you want to do to your partner or what you want them to do to you.

Be respectful: Make sure that both you and your partner are comfortable with sexting and that you're respecting their boundaries.

Using Dirty Talk to Set the Mood

Dirty talk can be a powerful tool for building arousal and intimacy during foreplay.

Here are some tips to get started:

Start off slow: Like with flirty texts, start off with some gentle teasing and suggestions. Gradually work your way up to more explicit language as both partners become more comfortable.

Pay attention to your partner's reactions: Watch your partner's reactions to see if what you're saying is turning them on or if they're feeling uncomfortable. Adjust accordingly.

Be respectful: As with any form of communication, be sure to respect your partner's boundaries and limitations. It's important to get consent before using explicit language or phrases.

Use descriptive language: Instead of using crude language, use descriptive language that paints a picture of what you're feeling, seeing, smelling, and experiencing in the moment.

Sharing Erotic Fantasies and Stories

Sharing erotic fantasies and stories can be a great way to enhance intimacy and build anticipation.

Here are some tips:

Start with a question: Ask your partner about their fantasies, and share your own in return. This can open up a dialogue about what turns you both on.

Cheryl Bach

Use descriptive language: Like with dirty talk, descriptive language can help bring your fantasies to life and make them more arousing.

Set the mood: To make the experience more immersive, set the mood by lighting candles, playing music, or visualizing the scene in your mind.

Be respectful: As with any form of communication, be sure to respect your partner's boundaries and limitations. It's important to get consent before sharing fantasies or stories that involve others.

Whispers and Moans

Incorporating whispers and moans can be a subtle yet highly effective way to heighten sexual tension during foreplay.

Here are some tips:

Whisper in your partner's ear: Bring your face close to your partner's ear and whisper suggestive messages or fantasies to them.

Moan softly: Make soft, low moans during foreplay to show your partner that you're enjoying what they're doing to you.

Use your breath: Use your breath to create sensations for your partner, like gently blowing on their ear or neck.

Pay attention to your partner's reactions: Like with dirty talk, it's important to pay attention to your partner's reactions and adjust accordingly. Some people may find whispers and moans highly arousing, while others may not.

In conclusion, verbal communication can be a powerful tool for building intimacy and arousal during foreplay. Techniques like flirty texts and sexting, dirty talk, sharing erotic fantasies and stories, and whispers and moans can all be highly effective ways to enhance your sexual experience.

Remember to always respect your partner's boundaries and comfort level, and communicate openly to find out what works best for both of you. By incorporating different techniques and finding what works best for you and your partner, you'll be well on your way to a more satisfying and pleasurable foreplay experience.

Chapter V
Techniques for Sensual Teasing

Sensual teasing is a powerful way to create erotic tension during foreplay. Here, we'll explore some techniques for teasing your partner and building anticipation for the main event.

Seductive Striptease

A seductive striptease can be a highly effective way to turn your partner on and build anticipation for what's to come.

Here are some tips:

Set the mood: Before you start the striptease, set the mood with lighting, music, and other elements that create a sensual atmosphere.

Slow it down: Take your time as you remove your clothing, and make sure to maintain eye contact with your partner throughout.

Be playful: Add some playful elements, like tossing your clothes in your partner's direction or using a prop like a feather boa or lap dance chair.

Incorporate movement: Don't be afraid to incorporate movement into your striptease, like twirling or dancing as you remove clothing. This can add an extra level of sensuality and excitement.

Cheryl Bach

Playing Hard-to-Get

Playing hard-to-get can be a powerful way to create erotic tension during foreplay.

Here are some tips:

Start slow: Don't give in to your partner's advances right away. Instead, start slow by gently teasing or playfully pushing them away.

Use body language: Use your body language to communicate that you're interested, but not quite ready to give in yet. Lean in close, touch them lightly, but then pull away.

Build up the anticipation: As you continue to play hard-to-get, build up the anticipation by whispering suggestive messages or giving subtle hints about what's to come.

Finally giving in: When you're ready to give in, do it all at once. This sudden change from playing hard-to-get to full-on passion can be incredibly arousing and exciting for your partner.

Using BDSM Techniques for Erotic Tension

BDSM techniques can be a highly effective way to create erotic tension during foreplay.

Here are some tips:

Start light: If you're new to BDSM, start with lighter techniques like bondage or sensory deprivation. As you become more comfortable, you can explore more intense techniques.

Communicate openly: BDSM requires a high level of communication and trust between partners. Talk openly about your boundaries and limitations, and establish a safeword so either partner can stop the action at any time.

Use sensory play: Sensory play is a common BDSM technique that involves using different sensations like touch, sound, and temperature to create erotic tension. Incorporate sensory play into your foreplay by using things like feathers, ice, or hot wax to surprise and stimulate your partner.

Explore power dynamics: BDSM is often about exploring power dynamics, so don't be afraid to experiment with dominant and submissive roles. This can add an extra level of excitement and anticipation to your play.

Sensory Deprivation and Temperature Play

Sensory deprivation and temperature play are two BDSM techniques that can be used to create erotic tension during foreplay.

Here are some tips:

Sensory Deprivation: Sensory deprivation involves removing certain senses like sight or hearing to heighten others. Blindfolding your partner or using earmuffs to block out sound can be highly effective for creating erotic tension during foreplay.

Temperature Play: Temperature play involves using hot or cold sensations to stimulate and tease the body. Here are some tips to incorporate temperature play into your foreplay:

Start slow: When using temperature play on your partner, start with a mild sensation and gradually get more intense as your partner becomes more aroused.

Use safe materials: It's important to use safe materials when incorporating temperature play into your foreplay. Never use anything that could cause serious injury or burns.

Experiment with different sensations: Try experimenting with different sensations, like using ice cubes, hot wax, or massage candles to add an extra level of excitement to your play.

Pay attention to your partner's reactions: As with any BDSM technique, it's important to pay attention to your partner's reactions and adjust accordingly. Don't continue with a sensation if your partner seems uncomfortable or in pain.

In conclusion, sensual teasing is an important part of foreplay and can be the key to unlocking incredible sexual pleasure. By incorporating seductive stripteases, playing hard-to-get, using BDSM techniques, and exploring sensory deprivation and temperature play, you can create erotic tension and anticipation for both you and your partner. Try experimenting with these techniques to find what works best for you and your partner, and enjoy the heightened pleasure and excitement that comes with sensual teasing during foreplay.

Chapter VI
Intimate Adventures in Advanced Foreplay

Foreplay is often an essential aspect of sexual pleasure, and there are countless techniques that you can incorporate into your routine to take things to the next level. In this chapter, we'll be exploring some advanced foreplay techniques that will help add a touch of passion, excitement, and intimacy to your sex life.

Tantric Sex Techniques for Extended Foreplay

Tantric sex is a practice that has been around for centuries, and it is focused on promoting intimacy and connection between partners. When practiced as part of your foreplay routine, it can help to take things to a deeper, more sensual level.

Here are some tantric sex techniques you can use:

Eye-gazing: Take a few minutes to look deeply into your partner's eyes without speaking. This can help to build intimacy and connection before you even start touching each other.

Breathwork: Syncing your breath with your partner's can help create a sense of unity and intimacy. Try sitting or lying down facing each other and focus on inhaling and exhaling together.

Sensual touch: Take the time to explore each other's bodies with slow and deliberate touches. Focus on the sensations you feel and try to stay present in the moment.

Tantric massage: This is a type of massage that focuses on stimulating erogenous zones and promoting relaxation and pleasure. Use sensual oils or lotions and take the time to explore each other's bodies in a slow and intimate way.

Bondage Techniques and Props

For some couples, adding elements of BDSM into their foreplay can be both exciting and empowering.

Here are some bondage techniques and props you can try:

Handcuffs: Using handcuffs can help to create a sense of power dynamic in your relationship, allowing one partner to take control and the other to submit. Start by applying the cuffs to the wrists and build up the tension as the foreplay progresses.

Blindfolds: Blindfolding your partner can help to heighten their senses as they are unable to see what is coming next. Try exploring different sensations with them, such as ice cubes or feathers.

Rope-play: This technique involves using ropes to tie up your partner in a way that accentuates their features, creating an intricate and beautiful pattern. It creates a sense of vulnerability and can be very sensual when done correctly.

Using Sex Toys Creatively as Part of Foreplay

Sex toys can provide unique sensations and add an extra level of excitement to your foreplay routine.

Here are some ways you can use them creatively:

Vibrators: Use a vibrator to stimulate your partner's erogenous zones, like the clitoris or nipples. You can also

Cheryl Bach

use it on yourself during mutual masturbation to intensify the experience.

Dildos: Incorporate a dildo into your foreplay by using it on your partner or yourself. Try experimenting with different sizes and shapes to find what works best for you.

Butt plugs: These toys can be used to stimulate the anus and prostate, which can create intense sensations. Use plenty of lube and start slowly.

Cock rings: These are worn around the base of the penis and can help to maintain an erection for longer, allowing for extended pleasure during foreplay.

Sex Games and Role Play

Sex games and role play are great ways to add an element of fun and playfulness to your foreplay routine.

Here are some ideas:

Strip poker: This classic game can be a great way to build up sexual tension and anticipation between you and your partner.

Truth or Dare: Use this game to explore each other's fantasies and desires in a playful and non-judgmental way.

Teacher/Student: This role play can be a fun way to explore power dynamics in the bedroom. Try switching roles to keep things interesting.

Naughty nurse/Patient: Dress up in sexy costumes and use props like a stethoscope or thermometer to create an immersive experience.

Cheryl Bach

In conclusion, foreplay is an essential aspect of sexual pleasure, and incorporating these advanced techniques into your routine can help to take things to the next level of intimacy, passion, and excitement with your partner. Try experimenting with different techniques and find what works best for you and your relationship.

Remember that communication is key, and always make sure that both partners are comfortable and consenting before incorporating any new techniques into your foreplay routine. Remember to have fun, be creative, and enjoy the journey of exploring each other's bodies and desires. By doing so, you'll create a deeper, more intimate, and satisfying sexual connection with your partner.

Chapter VII
Tips for Better Foreplay

Foreplay is an essential aspect of sexual intimacy that helps build excitement, arousal, and pleasure. Often, people make the mistake of rushing into sex without giving importance to foreplay, which can lead to unsatisfying and dull sexual experiences. In this chapter, we will be discussing some tips to improve your foreplay game and make it more intense and exciting.

Creating a Safe and Open Environment for Communication

One of the most crucial aspects of foreplay is establishing open and honest communication with your partner. Everyone has unique sexual preferences and desires.

Therefore, it's essential to create a safe space where both partners can openly communicate their needs and wants. Creating an environment where there's no room for judgment or shame will encourage both partners to express their sexual desires freely.

It's best to create an atmosphere where both partners can share their thoughts and feelings. Allow your partner to open up about what they enjoy during foreplay and what areas they'd like you to focus on more. Listening actively and without any form of judgment is key. Regular check-ins and conversations about desires will ensure that both partners remain comfortable throughout the entire experience.

Listening to Your Partner's Needs and Desires

Foreplay isn't a one-size-fits-all activity, and people have different ideas and preferences. Therefore, it's crucial to listen to your partner's needs and desires to ensure they are satisfied. It's not just about getting your partner ready for sex, as much as it is about increasing the intensity of the sexual experience.

Listen to your partner's verbal cues and non-verbal cues during the foreplay session--it's an excellent way to gauge how you're doing. Try to match their rhythm and pace as well as adjusting to their body language and sounds to ensure maximum pleasure. Note that everyone's needs and desires differ, and it's highly recommended to engage in active and open communication to create the best experience for you and your partner.

Being Creative and Experimental in Your Foreplay Techniques

Foreplay doesn't have to be limited to the basic techniques we all know. Being adventurous and trying out new things can bring excitement to your bedroom. Explore different techniques and allow yourselves to embrace creativity and experimentation. As stated earlier, everyone's preferences are diverse, what might work for one person may not necessarily work for another. Therefore, think outside the box and try out new techniques during foreplay--new positions, toys, and props. You never know what may excite both of you!

Prioritizing Pleasure for Both Partners

Foreplay isn't just about preparing your partner for sex; it's a shared experience of mutual pleasure. Both partners should feel equally involved, and the focus should be on giving pleasure as much as receiving it. Remember to prioritize your partner's pleasure throughout the entire experience. Focus on exploring their body, discovering their sweet spots and finding out what techniques turn them on the most. This will help you to create an intimate bond with your partner while giving them maximum pleasure.

Cheryl Bach

In conclusion, Foreplay isn't optional- it's an essential part of sexual intimacy that can make all the difference in creating truly pleasurable sex. Remember, everyone's needs and desires differ, so it's useful to communicate openly with your partner about what you both like and don't like. Listening to one another's needs, being creative and experimental with techniques, prioritizing mutual pleasure and creating a safe environment for open communication are all key ways to take your foreplay to the next level. These tips will help you discover new ways of improving intimacy in your sexual encounters and, ultimately, enhance everyone's pleasure.

Remember to start slow and work your way up to more advanced techniques that you both enjoy. Don't forget that exploration should be fun and enjoyable—never a chore or a source of anxiety. By using these tips, you can make foreplay a pleasurable and exciting part of your sex life!

Chapter VIII
Conclusion

Foreplay is an integral part of sexual intimacy between partners. It is not just something to tick off a checklist before sex, but it is the foundation of sexual pleasure and satisfaction. The right kind of foreplay can help you increase your emotional and physical connection with your partner. With so many benefits, it is only natural that foreplay should always be a priority in your sexual relationship.

Throughout this book, we have introduced you to the most sizzling hot foreplay tips, tricks and ideas that you can experiment with to enhance your sexual life. Implementing these ideas will result in a more passionate, fulfilling, and stimulating encounter with your partner. In effect, you may have discovered a raft of new possibilities for you and your lover to enjoy.

However, we must emphasize that there are no hard and fast rules about foreplay. It's essential to remember that each person is unique, and what works for one couple may not work for another. Therefore, you are encouraged to explore your own sexuality with your partner and try new things to determine what works best for you both.

It's also crucial to affirm the importance of foreplay in building intimacy and enhancing your overall sex life. Many couples often neglect foreplay in their sexual encounters, overlooking the fact that it is an essential component of sexual satisfaction. By prioritizing foreplay, you are nurturing your physical and emotional connection with your partner, helping to create a more fulfilling sexual relationship, and expressing your love non-verbally.

Finally, we must always prioritize communication and consent when engaging in foreplay or any form of sexual interaction with our partners. It is important to verbally and non-verbally communicate your desires, limits, and boundaries while also respecting those of your partner. Consent is crucial in both establishing and maintaining trust, respect, and healthy sexual relationships. It enables individuals to express their boundaries freely without fear of being shamed, guilted, or shunned. Additionally, communication helps build deeper intimacy with your partner by fostering trust, vulnerability, and openness.

In conclusion, foreplay is a vital aspect of sexual pleasure, and you have learned several exciting ideas and techniques to take your foreplay to the next level. We hope this guide has provided you with useful insights, tools, and techniques to help you improve your sex life with your partner. Remember always to be honest, respectful, and open with your partner while exploring the importance of foreplay in your relationship. With the right mindset and attitude, you can use foreplay to create deeper emotional intimacy and enhance your sexual satisfaction with your partner.

www.ingramcontent.com/pod-product-compliance
Lightning Source LLC
Chambersburg PA
CBHW051702250726
48653CB00007B/2805